# EMPATHY JOURNAL: A BOOK FOR KIDS

## This Journal Belongs to:

_____

# EMPATHY JOURNAL

## A BOOK FOR KIDS

### Prompts to Build Compassion and Understand the Feelings of Others

Kelley Stevens, LMFT

callisto
publishing
an imprint of Sourcebooks

To Max, the kindest kid I know. Love, Mom

Copyright © 2022 by Callisto Publishing LLC
Cover and internal design © 2022 by Callisto Publishing LLC
sceptical cactus / Creative Market
Author photo courtesy of Alex Lydia Photography
Interior and Cover Designer: Stephanie Sumulong
Art Producer: Melissa Malinowsky
Editor: Maxine Marshall
Production Editor: Jael Fogle
Production Manager: Riley Hoffman

Published by Callisto Publishing LLC C/O Sourcebooks LLC
P.O. Box 4410, Naperville, Illinois 60567-4410
(630) 961-3900
callistopublishing.com

Printed in the United States of America.

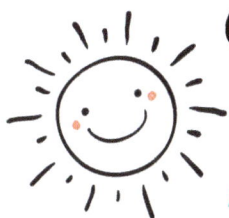

# Contents

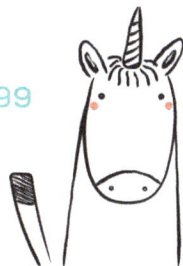

# A Note for Grown-Ups

Empathy means noticing other people's feelings and how they make us feel in turn. When your child uses empathy to imagine what it is like to be someone else, they learn to appreciate others' differences and develop strong interpersonal skills. As your child works through this journal, I invite you to focus on modeling empathetic behavior for them. Children learn by observing, and you have the opportunity to set a powerful example. Help your child apply the lessons from this journal by practicing and discussing empathy. You'll find a "Superpower Practice" in each section to help your child apply empathy skills to their daily lives.

There's no right or wrong time to use this journal—build the habit into your routine whenever it feels good for you and your child. This book should serve as a fun launching point for more discussions about empathy and kindness. You might consider bringing it on long car rides or doing a couple pages together before bed as your child is reflecting on their day.

# Welcome to Your Journal

Welcome to your new journal! This journal is full of fun and learning. It is made for kids just like you. Whether you are feeling busy or sleepy, or if you live in the city or by the beach, I have created this journal for you!

My name is Kelley Stevens. I help kids and families build empathy and kindness. Empathy is important in my life. It helps me understand my feelings and the feelings of my friends. Empathy also helps me imagine what other people might be seeing or thinking. This journal will help you explore empathy in your own life. It will help you understand your feelings, enjoy people's differences, and be a good friend. Let's get started!

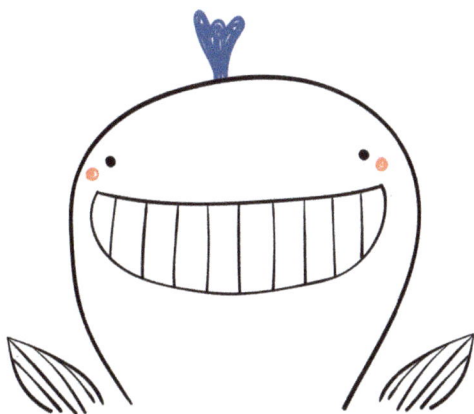

## What Is Empathy?

Empathy helps you picture what it is like to be someone else. Empathy means noticing what other people are feeling. It also means noticing how other people's feelings make you feel.

Has your friend ever forgotten their lunch at home? Did you notice how sad they felt when they didn't have a lunch to eat? Did it make you feel sad, too? That is empathy!

Empathy helps you be a better friend. Empathy helps you see all the different ways that people feel. This journal will help you connect to other people. It will also help you understand your own thoughts and feelings.

Empathy is a superpower! It helps us do great things. You can practice empathy even when you aren't using this journal. Empathy is something we can practice all the time with the people around us.

## How to Use This Journal

Guess what? You can use this journal any way you want. You can write and draw in it anytime. There are no rules! You can write while you are listening to music, hanging out in your room, or having a yummy snack. You can share this journal with a friend, parent, or trusted adult. Remember to always ask for help if you need it. Learning about empathy will be fun.

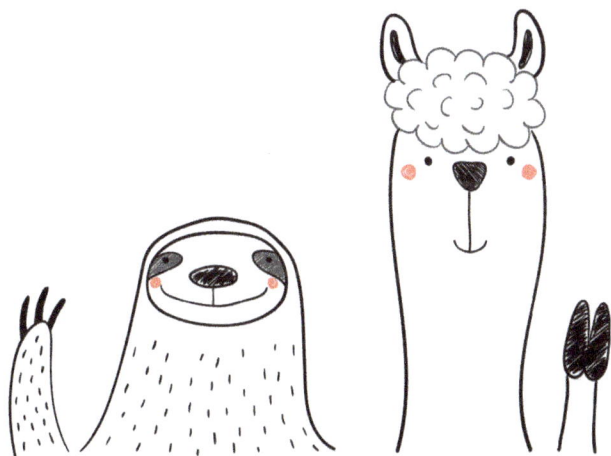

# THE BIG WORLD OF FEELINGS

**W**elcome! In this section, you will learn all about your feelings. How do you feel when something doesn't go the way you want it to? How do you feel when you see your friends? We will explore those emotions together. We will also discover more about the feelings of other people. You will learn how to understand other people's feelings. Understanding feelings helps us be a super friend, a good listener, and a kind family member.

What does it mean to feel angry?

_____

_____

_____

_____

What color would you match with the feeling
of anger? What color would you match with
feeling happy?

_____

_____

_____

_____

What is a good way to tell someone you
understand how they feel?

_____

_____

_____

# Faces and Feelings

Faces give us clues to know what someone else is feeling. Someone who is happy might be laughing. Someone who is sad might be looking down or crying. Faces can tell us if our friends are angry, sad, or afraid. Draw a face to match each feeling word.

| | |
|---|---|
| **Sad** | **Angry** |
| **Happy** | **Afraid** |

Remember a time when you noticed that a friend felt sad. What were they doing that told you they were feeling sad?

_____

_____

_____

Write about a time you felt angry. How did your tummy feel when you were angry? How did your head feel when you were angry?

_____

_____

_____

When was the last time you felt very excited? How did your body feel when you were excited?

_____

_____

_____

# My Feelings and My Body

We feel our feelings in our minds and in our bodies. Our bodies give us clues about how we are feeling. It is important to learn how your feelings feel in your body. For each event, write how your tummy or mouth feels.

| EVENT | HOW MY TUMMY FEELS | HOW MY MOUTH FEELS |
|---|---|---|
| My best friend gives me a birthday card. | | |
| I drop my sandwich on the floor. | | |
| It is my first day at a new school. | | |
| My family is going to an amusement park. | | |

What does it mean to feel lonely?

_____

_____

_____

_____

Have you ever seen someone get angry? How did
you feel when you saw they were angry?

_____

_____

_____

_____

Imagine you are an octopus. How would your
tentacles move if you were relaxed? How would
your tentacles move if you were excited?

_____

_____

_____

# Colors Make Us Feel

Colors can make us feel different feelings. Sometimes people feel happy when they see the color yellow or sad when they see the color blue. Can you think of some colors that make you feel happy? Draw a picture of a time when you felt happy. Use colors that make you feel happy right now.

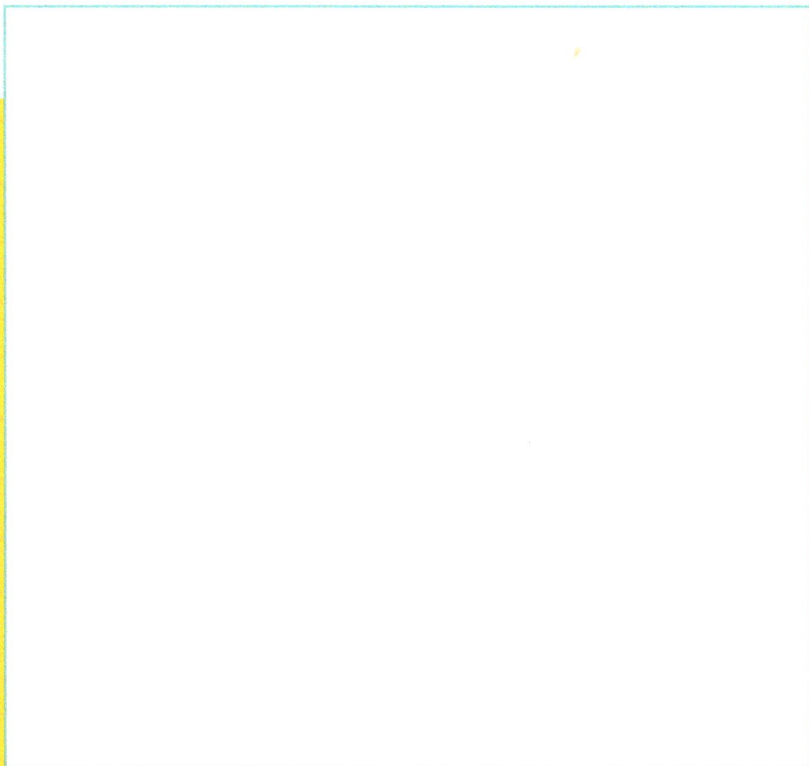

Write about a time when you saw a friend who felt embarrassed. What happened to make them feel embarrassed? What did their face look like?

_____

_____

_____

_____

How does your mind feel when you are late for school? How does your body feel when you are late for school?

_____

_____

_____

Why is it important to notice when a friend feels lonely?

_____

_____

_____

## Feelings and Actions

Sometimes our friends' actions give us clues about how they are feeling. For example, someone who is angry might yell. Someone who is calm might sit still and take big breaths. Let's practice matching actions with feelings. Circle all the actions that tell you that your friend is happy.

My friend is smiling.

# My friend is laughing.

My friend is crying.

# My friend is playing.

My friend is looking down at their feet.

# My friend is telling a funny joke.

My friend is making mean faces.

Imagine you are a little puppy. How would you show the other puppies you are lonely?

_____

_____

_____

If your tummy hurts or your head aches, how would you tell your parents or family members about it? Try to use words that help them imagine what you feel like.

_____

_____

_____

Think about how you are feeling right now. How does your tummy feel? How do your arms and legs feel?

_____

_____

_____

How do you feel when a friend gets a new toy but you don't get one?

_____

_____

_____

_____

How do you feel when you find out two of your friends had a playdate without you?

_____

_____

_____

_____

What feelings do you feel on your birthday? Do you feel that way any other time of the year?

_____

_____

_____

# Feelings Are All Around Us

Feelings are caused by the things you see and by the things that happen in your life. Think about it: When you see your best friend, you feel happy or excited to play. If one of your toys breaks, you might feel angry. Read each example and think about how it makes you feel. Write down a word to describe that feeling.

| SOMETHING I SEE | HOW IT MAKES ME FEEL |
|---|---|
| A broken toy | |
| A giant cookie | |
| A puppy | |
| A friend waiting for me at the playground | |
| A balloon | |

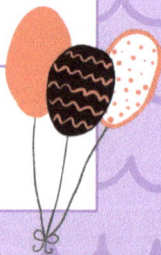

Think of a time when you noticed a friend feeling nervous. What did their face look like?

_____

_____

_____

_____

What are two feelings you might feel if a friend asks you to break a rule?

_____

_____

_____

What is one good way to make up after you argue with a friend? Have you ever done this in real life? If so, write about it here.

_____

_____

_____

Remember a time you felt proud. How did your body feel?

_____

_____

_____

Write about how your body feels when you are nervous. What about when you are excited? Do those feelings feel similar in your body, or different?

_____

_____

_____

What is your favorite feeling? Why?

_____

_____

_____

# Feelings in the World

Different events can cause us to feel different feelings. For example, on your birthday you might feel excited, happy, or joyful. Draw how you feel when these events happen.

| | |
|---|---|
| **You forgot to bring your homework to school.** | **You dropped your sandwich in the dirt.** |
| **You made a new friend at recess.** | **You scored a soccer goal.** |

Imagine you could visit nice aliens on a planet far away. They don't speak your language. How would you talk to them without using words? How would you use your hands and face to show them you are their friend?

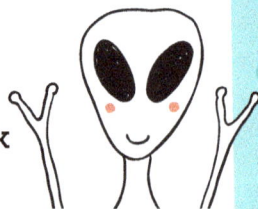

_____

_____

_____

Is it easy or difficult to say you are sorry? Write about a time you told someone you were sorry.

_____

_____

_____

How does your body feel when you are happy?

_____

_____

_____

# Caring for Others

Everyone has feelings. Feelings are a special part of being human. We can show other people we care for them by showing them we care about their feelings. Caring for other people's feelings is an important part of empathy. Place a check mark next to all the reasons it is important to care about other people's feelings.

It is important to care about other people's feelings because:

☐ It shows them I care about them.

☐ It helps them pick out a Halloween costume.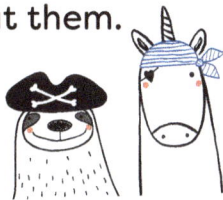

☐ It makes them feel loved.

☐ It helps them get really good at soccer.

☐ It makes it easier to get what I want.

☐ It makes them care about my feelings, too.

Imagine you are a little kitten who hurt his paw. What are you feeling?

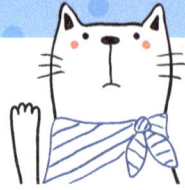

_____

_____

_____

A baby turtle can't find her mom. How do you think the turtle feels?

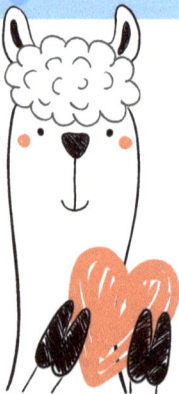

_____

_____

_____

Think of a time you showed kindness to an animal. What did you do?

_____

_____

_____

## Feelings Fish

If you were a little fish swimming in the sea, what do you imagine you would be feeling? What colors would your scales be? Draw a picture of your fish here. Use colors that match your feelings.

Have you ever felt confused at school? How did your stomach feel when you were confused?

_____

_____

_____

_____

What is your least-favorite feeling? Why?

_____

_____

_____

_____

Make a list of all the feelings you can think of.

_____

_____

_____

_____

_____

# Understanding Feelings

Sometimes it is hard to know what our friends and family are feeling. We can look at their words, faces, and bodies for clues. Let's practice matching people's faces and bodies with their feelings. Draw a line to match each sentence to a feeling word.

| | |
|---|---|
| Sydney is crying. | Excited |
| Juliet has a big smile on her face. | Angry |
| Max's face is red, and he's pouting. | Sad |
| Aiden is jumping up and down. | Happy |
| Avery is yawning. | Tired |

Imagine you are a bird flying in the sky. What feelings might you have while you are flying?

_____

_____

_____

Imagine you are on a submarine exploring the ocean. How do you feel? What do you see?

_____

_____

_____

Imagine it is the first day of school, and your friend is nervous to meet your new teacher. What do their eyebrows do to show they are nervous? What does their mouth look like?

_____

_____

_____

# SUPERPOWER PRACTICE: TALKING TO A TRUSTED ADULT

The next time you feel sad or lonely, try talking to a trusted adult. When you speak with them, follow these steps to share how you are feeling.

**1.** Say, "I feel _____."

**2.** Tell them what made you feel this way.

**3.** Tell them how they can help.

Can you think of a time you talked to a trusted adult when you were feeling sad? Write about that here.

_____

_____

_____

_____

_____

_____

_____

# PUTTING ON SOMEONE ELSE'S SHOES

Everyone has different feelings. This makes everyone unique and special. Empathy helps you notice how other people's feelings are different from your own. Empathy helps you imagine you are wearing someone else's shoes. (But not their real shoes. That could be smelly!) Putting yourself in someone else's shoes means understanding what it is like to be them.

It is easiest to hear other people's feelings when we are calm. What is one thing you can do to help your body feel calm?

_____

_____

_____

_____

Describe what your body feels like when you are relaxed.

_____

_____

_____

_____

Is it possible to feel relaxed when you are with your friends who feels excited?

_____

_____

_____

# Knowing Your Family's Hearts

Empathy means feeling what is inside someone else's heart. When we feel empathy for a family member, we feel what they might be feeling or thinking. Inside the heart, draw something that would make a person in your family feel calm and relaxed.

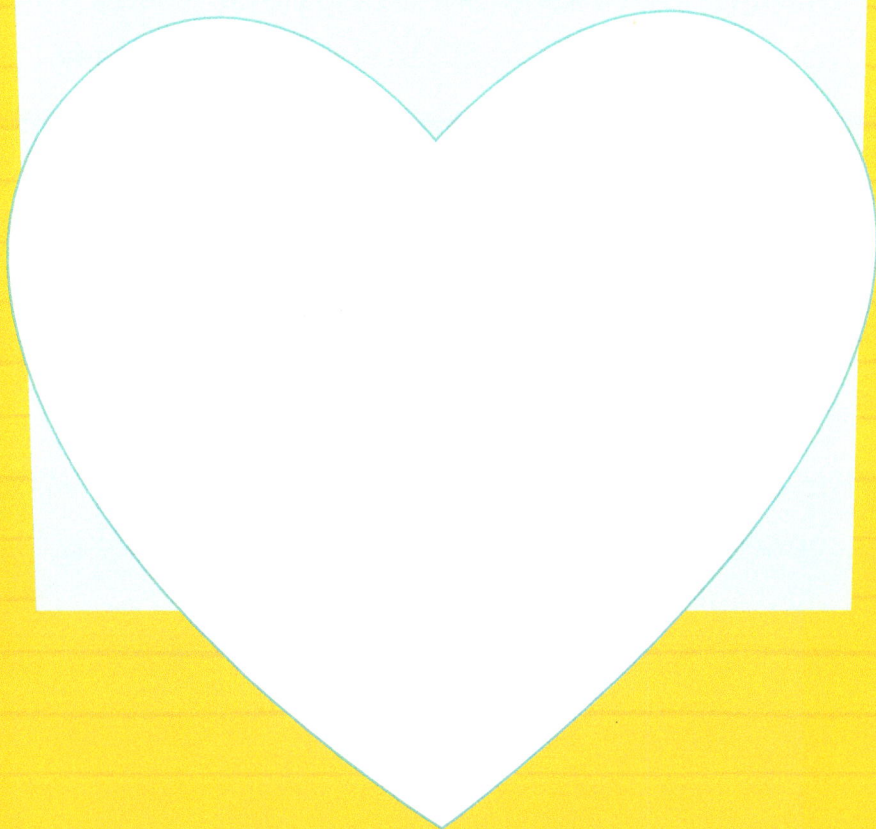

Write about a time you felt sad while your friends felt happy.

_____

_____

_____

If someone you know was feeling joyful, what is one sign you would notice that would tell you they are feeling joy?

_____

_____

_____

Imagine you see a puppy who is left out by his brothers and sisters. What do you think the puppy might be feeling?

_____

_____

_____

# Seeing Things Differently

People think and feel different things. This is what makes us all special. For each idea, write down what you think and then write down what a friend might think about the idea.

| | WHAT I THINK | WHAT MY FRIEND THINKS |
|---|---|---|
| What is the best flavor of ice cream? | | |
| What is the most fun game to play during recess? | | |
| What is your favorite thing to do on the weekend? | | |
| Do you like to go to bed early or stay up late? | | |

Do you and your friend always agree?

_____

Is it okay for you and your friend to think differently?

_____

_____

Imagine how your parent or guardian might feel if you lied to them. Have you ever lied to your parent or guardian? How did lying make you feel?

_____

_____

_____

Imagine a kid at school is being called mean names on the playground. How do you think the kid is feeling?

_____

_____

_____

Pretend you are a frog who got stuck on a log in the middle of a deep river. How would you feel?

_____

_____

_____

# My Favorite and Your Favorite

Draw a picture of your favorite food. Then draw a picture of your friend's favorite food. Are the foods the same or different?

| MY FAVORITE FOOD | MY FRIEND'S FAVORITE FOOD |
| --- | --- |
|  |  |

Imagine you watch a movie with a friend, and you hate the movie. Your friend loves the movie. What is one way you can kindly express the fact that you felt differently about the movie?

_____

_____

_____

How would one of your classmates feel if the teacher told them to stop talking during class? Has this ever happened to you? How did you feel?

_____

_____

_____

Think about how a friend would feel if they heard their parents arguing. Would they feel sad, lonely, or afraid? Or all three?

_____

_____

_____

# Calming Your Body

It is important to calm our bodies even when people around us are not calm. Fill in the blanks with ways that you can calm your body. Use ideas from the box or make up your own.

## IDEA BOX

Take a deep breath.

Draw a picture.

Talk to an adult I trust.

Think of something that makes me happy.

Touch my toes and wiggle my fingers.

Take a nap or a break.

1. When my friend is sad, I can do this to calm my body: _____

_____

2. When my teacher gets frustrated with another student, I can do this to calm my body:

_____

_____

3. When my parent or guardian is grumpy, I can do this to calm my body: _____

_____

Think about your favorite thing to eat for dinner. Is your favorite dinner the same as or different from your best friend's favorite dinner?

_____

_____

_____

Our world is beautiful because all people are unique. Gardens are the same way—they are wonderful because no two flowers are the same. Let's plant an imaginary garden! What colors of flowers would you plant in your garden?

_____

_____

How do you feel when you go to a friend's house to play? How do you think your friends feel when they come to your house to play?

_____

_____

Do you think that all puppies like to play outside? Or would some puppies rather stay inside and snuggle on the couch?

_____

_____

_____

A little sloth is learning how to climb trees. She climbs high and is very proud! But when she looks around, she can't see her home anymore. How do you think the sloth feels?

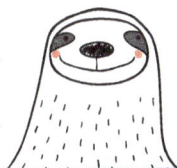

_____

_____

What is something you have never done before but want to try?

_____

_____

_____

# Different Days and Different Feelings

Read each of the stories that follow. Imagine what the animal is feeling and circle all the words that match their emotions.

A puppy is left alone in a house while his owners are at work and school. Circle all the feelings he might be feeling:

| | | |
|---|---|---|
| **Lonely** | **Hungry** | **Joyful** |
| **Tired** | **Happy** | **Excited** |
| | **Silly** | |

A young giraffe can't find her giraffe friends to play with. She is standing by a tree and looking for them. Circle all the feelings she might be feeling:

| | | |
|---|---|---|
| **Hungry** | **Lonely** | **Playful** |
| **Grumpy** | **Bored** | **Calm** |
| | **Scared** | |

A baby bird just found something yummy to eat, and he is eating while looking out at a big lake. Circle all the feelings he might be feeling:

| | | |
|---|---|---|
| **Worried** | **Excited** | **Loved** |
| **Happy** | **Hungry** | **Nervous** |
| | **Adventurous** | |

What is your favorite food to eat at lunchtime? Do you like to bring this food to school? What foods do your classmates like to eat at school?

_____

_____

_____

Imagine a classmate who is taller than everyone else. How do you think they feel as the tallest person in the class? Are there activities or sports that they might be great at because they are tall?

_____

_____

_____

Your friend wants to play catch at recess. You want to go on the swings. What is one way you can compromise with your friend?

_____

_____

Do your friends' families celebrate holidays with different traditions than your family? Write down one thing that makes their celebrations unique.

_____

_____

_____

What is one thing that makes your family different from other families?

_____

_____

_____

Have you ever loved a book that your friends didn't enjoy?

_____

_____

_____

# My Family and Your Family

Draw a picture of your family. Then draw a picture of your friend's family. Don't forget the pets! Notice all the special things that make each of your families one of a kind.

| MY FAMILY | MY FRIEND'S FAMILY |
| --- | --- |
|  |  |

Do your friends enjoy playing any games that you don't like?

_____

_____

_____

_____

Imagine you are in a boat. What can you see from your boat? Is it different from what you can see right now?

_____

_____

_____

Your friend asks to borrow your favorite color marker. How does your body feel when you are asked to share?

_____

_____

_____

# Using Empathy

Let's practice using empathy. Read the situation and then answer the questions.

**Situation: Hudson broke his friend's toy by accident.**

How do you think Hudson is feeling? _____

_____

_____

Have you ever felt the way Hudson is feeling? Circle **YES** or **NO**

When? _____

_____

_____

When you felt this way, what helped you feel better?

_____

_____

What could you say to Hudson to help him feel better?

_____

_____

What does it mean to imagine yourself in someone else's shoes?

_____

_____

_____

Imagine you are a baby horse. All the other baby horses love eating carrots, but you like eating apples. How does it feel to like a snack that is different from the snack your friends like?

_____

_____

_____

Do all your friends love playing outside? Do you have some friends who prefer to play inside?

_____

_____

_____

## Putting On Someone Else's Shoes

Remember the idea of putting on someone else's shoes? That means imagining how it might feel to be that person. Think of a time when you "put on" your friend's shoes and understood what they were feeling. Draw a picture of that here. Use different colors to show the feelings you were feeling on that day.

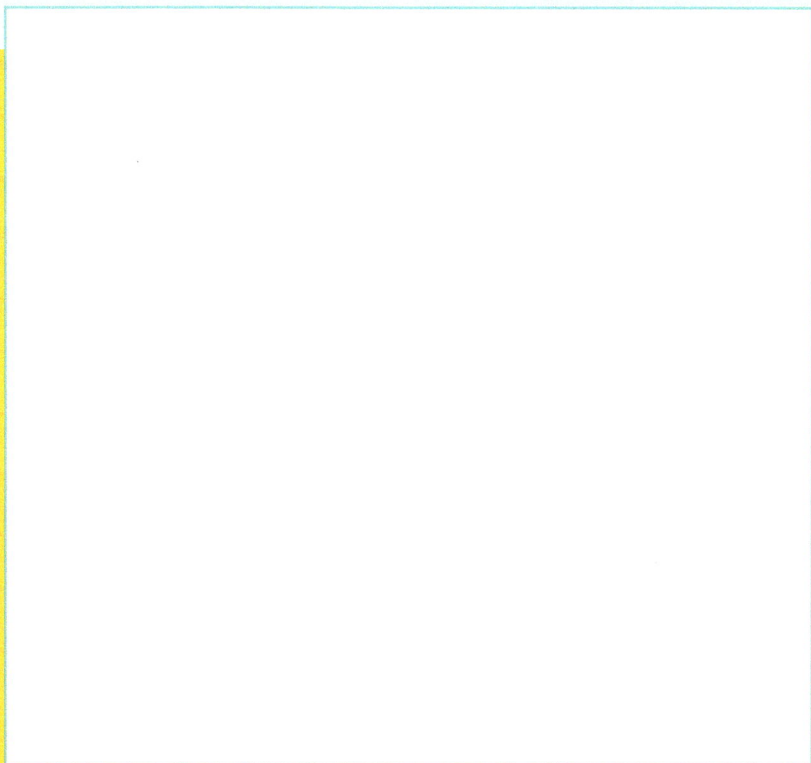

Your friend tells you they like a TV show that you didn't like. How do you respond?

_____

_____

_____

A friend tells you they love math. You really don't like math. What do you say to your friend about the subject?

_____

_____

_____

Imagine your friend is excited to watch a scary movie but you feel afraid. How do you tell your friend that you feel afraid?

_____

_____

_____

# What to Do When We Disagree

Sometimes our thoughts are not the same as other people's thoughts. Let's practice using empathy when we disagree. Read the story. Check off the ways Juan and Lena can use empathy to kindly disagree.

**Juan loves to watch animal shows on TV after school. Juan's sister, Lena, loves to watch cartoons. They have only one TV. Every afternoon, they argue about which show is the "best." They never agree, and the arguments often get so bad their parents take away their TV privileges. How can Juan and Lena work it out?**

☐ Continue to argue

☐ Hit each other

☐ Take turns with what show they will watch

☐ Talk kindly to each other

☐ Understand that they can have different ideas of which show is the best

☐ Pick a new show they both like

Your parent or guardian really likes listening to the news in the car, but you like to listen to music. What is a respectful way to tell them you want to listen to music?

_____

_____

What is one way that you can calm your body down when you are feeling overwhelmed?

_____

_____

Everyone learns differently. Some of us learn best by writing down our ideas, while some of us need breaks to wiggle our bodies to help us learn best. Write down what helps you learn. Then write down what you notice about how other people learn at your school.

_____

_____

# SUPERPOWER PRACTICE: CELEBRATING DIFFERENCE

Everyone is special and unique. We all think and feel different things. We can practice empathy in the real world by celebrating the differences we see.

The next time you notice someone who is different from you, try these things to show them you appreciate all the wonderful things that make them unique:

☐ Ask what they like to do for fun and ask if you can join them.

☐ Ask them to tell you something unique about themselves.

☐ Pause and just listen; it is okay if you don't know what to say.

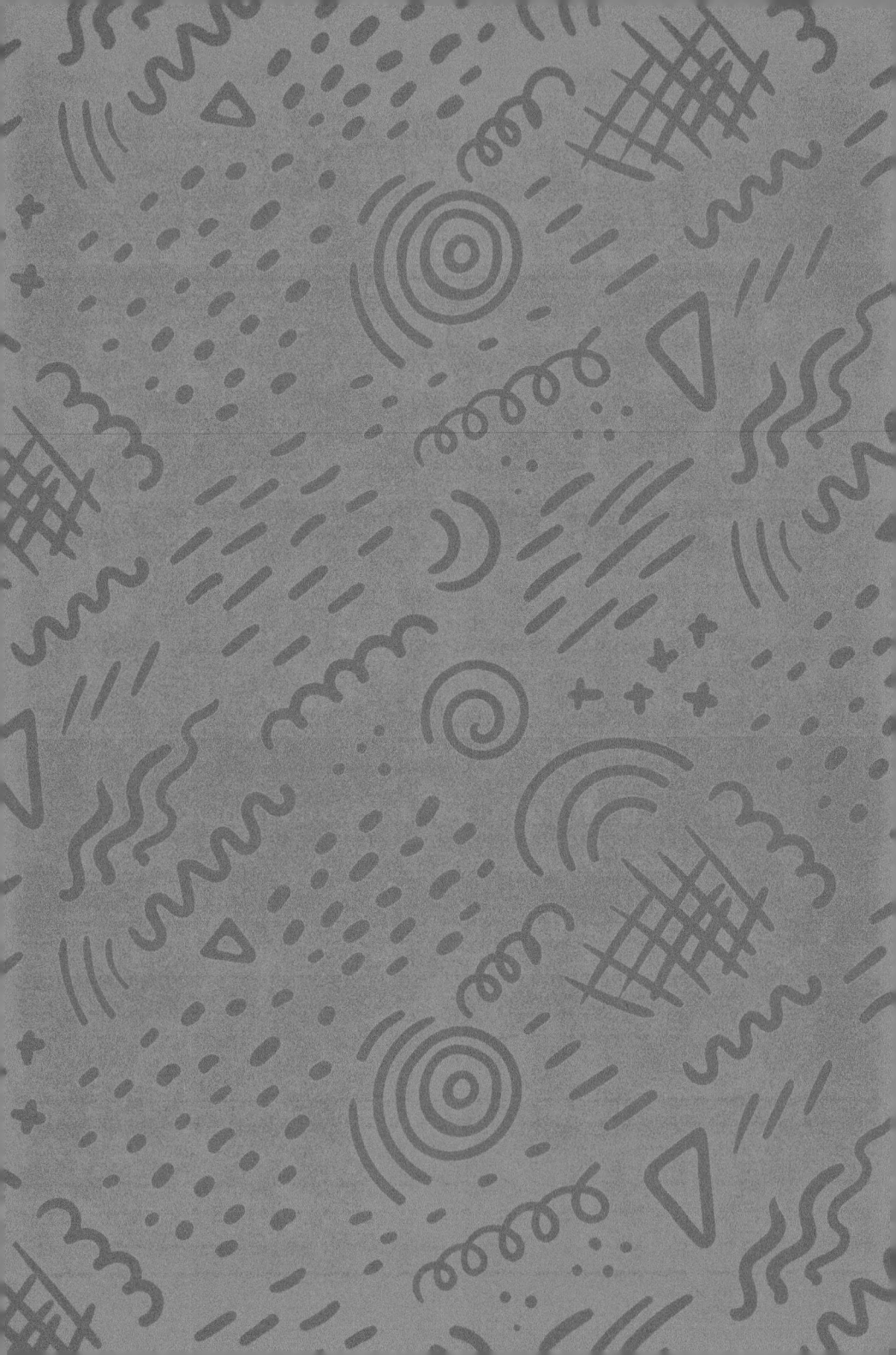

# A LITTLE KINDNESS GOES A LONG WAY

Did you know that showing a little bit of kindness can make someone feel a lot better? Let's practice showing care and kindness! You will learn how to be kind, caring, and compassionate toward others. Kindness can be actions, like helping your teacher clean the classroom. Or kindness can be words, like telling a friend how special they are. This journal is here to help you practice using kind actions and words.

What does it mean to be kind?

_____

_____

_____

_____

Write down three things you can do to help a friend who is sad.

_____

_____

_____

_____

What are three actions you can take when you see that a friend is being left out?

_____

_____

_____

_____

# Being Kind to the Planet

Draw a picture of yourself doing something to help the environment. Some ideas are planting a tree and picking up litter. Use one of these ideas or come up with your own.

What are two actions you can take to help a friend who is lonely? Write them down.

_____

_____

_____

Write about a time when you helped a friend who was worried. How did you help them?

_____

_____

_____

Imagine you are a duckling. Your brother duck is having a hard time swimming across the pond. What is one thing you can do to help him?

_____

_____

_____

## Showing Friends We Care

Being a good friend means understanding how our friends feel. It also means doing little things to show our friends we care about them. Circle all the things that make someone a good friend.

I listen when my friend is talking.

# I make fun of my friend.

I make eye contact when my friend is telling me something.

# I share my toys with my friend.

I ask my friend how they are feeling.

I leave my friend out when they want to play.

I ask my friend what games they want to play.

I ask my friend if they want a hug when they are sad.

I make mean faces at my friend.

Write down two things you can do to be helpful in your classroom.

_____

_____

_____

_____

Write about a time you showed kindness to a friend. What did you do?

_____

_____

_____

A new kid at summer camp hasn't made any friends yet. How do you think they are feeling? Write down one thing you can do to help them feel welcome.

_____

_____

_____

# Helpful Bears

Draw a picture of a bear helping a smaller bear in the forest. What are the bears' names?

How does it make you feel when you put away your toys after you play with them?

_____

_____

_____

Imagine you are sending your best friend a birthday card. What would you write in the birthday card?

_____

_____

_____

Write down three ways you can show kindness to a puppy.

_____

_____

_____

## Showing Kindness and Respect to Everyone

All people deserve to be treated with kindness. Read the story about Charlie. Then circle all the ways you can show kindness and respect to Charlie.

**Charlie is a seven-year-old boy. He loves to laugh and learn. When Charlie speaks, he sounds a little different than his friends, and it takes him longer to finish some tasks. Sometimes this makes Charlie feel frustrated and sad.**

We want to show Charlie kindness. Circle YES or NO to show whether a behavior is kind.

Make a kind face when you see him. **YES** or **NO**

Get to know him and be a friend to him. **YES** or **NO**

Make a mean face at him. **YES** or **NO**

Ask him if you can help with anything. **YES** or **NO**

Tell your friends lies about him. **YES** or **NO**

Learn what he likes to do and ask to join him. **YES** or **NO**

What does it mean to be a good listener? Can you describe a time when you were a good listener?

_____

_____

_____

What does it mean to be honest? Write about a time you were honest even though it was hard.

_____

_____

_____

What should you do if you are feeling angry and don't feel like being kind?

_____

_____

_____

We can be kind to plants and animals, just like we can be kind to people. What is one way you can help the environment?

_____

_____

_____

_____

What is one thing you can do to help make your classroom feel calm and peaceful?

_____

_____

_____

_____

Write about a time when you tried to make someone feel special. How did it make you feel?

_____

_____

_____

## Adults with Empathy

Did you know that many adults try to practice empathy? Some adults have jobs that help the people around them. Read the list of jobs. Write down one thing each job does to help other people.

Teacher: _____
_____

Nurse: _____
_____

Firefighter: _____
_____

Parent: _____
_____

Chef: _____
_____

Write down one action you do that makes other people smile.

_____

_____

_____

What is one good way to help your parents or family members? Have you ever done this in real life?

_____

_____

_____

_____

What is one action you can take to help a friend who feels sad because their dog is sick?

_____

_____

_____

Imagine there is a kid in your class who speaks slowly and sometimes forgets words. What is one way you can show them you are listening and you care about what they are saying?

_____

_____

_____

Who is the kindest person you know? What makes them so kind?

_____

_____

_____

You notice a piece of trash on the ground at the playground. What can you do with the trash?

_____

_____

_____

## Asking for Help

We all need help sometimes. You have people in your life, like friends, teachers, and family, who are there to help when you need it. Draw a picture of a time when you needed help from someone else. Use different colors to show what you were feeling when you needed help.

Is it easy or hard to help other people? What makes it easy or hard?

_____

_____

_____

All people make mistakes. What can you say to a friend who feels bad that they made a mistake?

_____

_____

_____

Imagine you are at your friend's birthday party. They got lots of presents. You are feeling jealous because it's not your birthday. What can you do to show you are still happy for your friend even though you feel jealous?

_____

_____

_____

# Expressing Gratitude

Learning to tell other people that we are thankful for them is an awesome way to show empathy and kindness. Fill in the blanks to practice gratitude.

A family member I am thankful for: _____

_____

A friend I am thankful for: _____

_____

A quality about myself I am thankful for: _____

_____

An animal I am thankful for: _____

_____

The next time I see _____ I will show them I am grateful for them by _____

_____

Who is the one person you are most grateful for?
Write down one thing you like about this person.

_____

_____

_____

Imagine you are a monkey in the jungle. One of
the other monkeys stole your banana. What can
you say to kindly ask for your banana back?

_____

_____

_____

Write down one way you can show kindness to an
elderly person.

_____

_____

_____

# Different Traditions

Draw a picture of a friend or neighbor whose family celebrates a different holiday from your family. Include things that make their holiday special, like delicious food or fun decorations.

Write down three things that always put you in a good mood.

_____

_____

_____

_____

What is one thing that you can do to show kindness to someone who annoys you?

_____

_____

_____

_____

What does it mean to be respectful? What is one way you can show respect to your teacher?

_____

_____

_____

# Empathy Bingo

Empathy is awesome! We can use our empathy in real life. After you complete an empathy activity, check it off. Complete all the actions in a row or column to win Empathy Bingo. Bonus challenge: Can you complete all 16 actions?

| | | | |
|---|---|---|---|
| Help someone before they ask. | Smile at a kid who often gets left out. | Ask a friend if they want a hug. | Offer to share school supplies with a classmate. |
| Compliment a friend on something they are good at. | Ask a friend how they are feeling. | Notice when your friend is feeling tired. | Share a toy without being asked. |
| Help your friend find a lost toy. | Help your teacher with a task at school. | Help a parent or family member clean up. | Do something nice for an animal (petting a dog, feeding a fish). |
| Get help for a friend who is hurt. | Offer to help your parent take out the trash. | Sit with someone who looks lonely. | Say thank you to a parent or family member. |

Does your family do anything special to help other people? If so, write about that here. If not, what is something that you would like to do with your family to help other people? Write about it here.

_____

_____

Imagine you are meeting someone from another country. You don't speak the same language. What can you do to greet them even though you don't understand each other?

_____

_____

Imagine a new kid just moved to your neighborhood. What can you do to make them feel welcome?

_____

_____

# SUPERPOWER PRACTICE: ACTS OF KINDNESS

Empathy helps us show kindness to our friends and family. Kindness means helping the people you care about. Write down the names of three people who are important to you. Then write down one thing you will do to show each of those people kindness this week.

| NAME | ACT OF KINDNESS |
|------|-----------------|
|      |                 |
|      |                 |
|      |                 |

## SECTION 4

# BEING THE BEST FRIEND YOU CAN BE

**Y**ou can use empathy every day to be kind to your friends and family. Your journal is here to help you practice. You will learn to listen, share, and work together so you can have the most fun with other people. Let's explore skills like using your words to set boundaries and sharing even when you don't want to. These skills will help you be a kind, respectful friend to everyone. Now practice being the best friend and family member you can be!

The student next to you in class is teasing your friend. What should you do?

_____

_____

_____

What should you do if someone tells you they don't want you to stand too close to them?

_____

_____

_____

Penny and Frankie love the same shows, listen to the same music, and dress the same way. But Penny hates pizza and Frankie loves pizza. What can Penny do to show she respects Frankie's choices?

_____

_____

_____

# Fun with Friends

Draw a picture of yourself doing each action.

**Saying "I'm sorry" to a friend**

**Sharing a toy with a friend**

**Playing my favorite game**

Write down something you love about your neighborhood. Now use your imagination and dream big! If you could add something to your neighborhood to make it better for everyone, what would it be?

_____

_____

Write down two ways you can show someone you are listening.

_____

_____

_____

Imagine you are playing on a soccer team with your friends. How do you become a good teammate? Write down three qualities that make a good teammate.

_____

_____

# Making Things Better

Our actions can make things worse or help make things better. In the following boxes, write down two things that can make the situations worse and two things that can make the situations better.

| When I'm having an argument with a friend . . . | |
| --- | --- |
| MAKES IT WORSE | MAKES IT BETTER |
| | |
| | |

| When I'm helping my family pick up toys . . . | |
| --- | --- |
| MAKES IT WORSE | MAKES IT BETTER |
| | |
| | |

| When I am riding in the car with my family on the way to school . . . | |
| --- | --- |
| MAKES IT WORSE | MAKES IT BETTER |
| | |
| | |

Two kids at the park want to use the same swing. What is one way they can work out this problem?

_____

_____

_____

What does it mean to be honest with your friends? Write about one time when you were honest in your friendship but you were very tempted to tell a lie.

_____

_____

_____

Imagine your parent or guardian asked you to wait a minute before they can help you. How does your body feel when you are asked to wait?

_____

_____

_____

## Weekend Fun

Draw a picture of your favorite thing to do on the weekend with your family. Use different colors to show the way you feel when you are doing the activity.

What is one compliment you can give a friend? How do you think this compliment would make them feel inside?

_____

_____

_____

_____

Do you have a nickname? Who calls you by your nickname?

_____

_____

_____

_____

Whom do you share your secrets and feelings with?

_____

_____

_____

## Setting Boundaries

A boundary is a simple rule that you make. A boundary helps other people know how to treat you. Boundaries help you tell people what is okay and what is not okay for them to do to you. Look at the list of boundaries that follows. Check off the boundaries you would like to use in your life. You can use these words to set boundaries with others or come up with your own words.

☐ I don't feel comfortable talking about that.

☐ I don't like when you speak to me that way.

☐ You are standing too close to me. Please give me some space.

☐ I don't like when you call me that.

☐ That is making me feel uncomfortable. Please stop.

Who is allowed to know where you live and your address?

_____

_____

_____

Does it ever feel difficult to share your toys? What can you tell yourself when you feel annoyed about sharing a toy?

_____

_____

_____

Write down one way you can show someone that you are thankful for them.

_____

_____

_____

Imagine you are very tired but your friend wants to run around the playground. What can you say to your friend to let them know you need a break?

_____

_____

Imagine your sibling said something that hurt your feelings. Write down a good way to tell them you don't like what they said. How does it make you feel to think about saying it?

_____

_____

Pretend you are a fuzzy monkey! You see another monkey making an awesome jump from one tree to another. What is one thing you can say to that monkey to celebrate their success?

_____

_____

# Sharing Is Caring

Sometimes sharing feels difficult. You might not always feel like you want to share, but sharing helps us be better friends. In the following boxes, write down four things that you find easy to share and four things that are hard to share.

| EASY TO SHARE | HARD TO SHARE |
|---|---|
|  |  |
|  |  |
|  |  |
|  |  |

**Bonus!** Write down one thing in each list that you will share with a friend very soon.

_____

_____

_____

Have you ever felt uncomfortable when someone was standing too close to you? What is something you can say when someone is standing closer to you than you want?

_____

_____

_____

Imagine you have a friend who gets overwhelmed by loud noises. What is one activity you can do with them that isn't loud?

_____

_____

_____

Have you ever asked a friend or trusted adult for help? Write about that here.

_____

_____

_____

Have you ever talked very loudly in a quiet place? How did you feel when you spoke louder than everyone else?

_____

_____

_____

Imagine one of your friends hurt your feelings. How can you let them know they said something that hurt you?

_____

_____

_____

Write down three ways you can work together with your friends to build a fort.

_____

_____

_____

## Feeling Safe

A baby rabbit is afraid because a big snake is coming too close. Draw a picture of the baby rabbit and the snake. Add something to your picture to help the rabbit feel safe.

Why is it important to say you are sorry when you hurt someone's feelings?

_____

_____

_____

_____

Have you ever had to take turns using a toy? How did it feel to share a toy with a friend or sibling?

_____

_____

_____

_____

Close your eyes and send a positive thought to a friend. Write down what your positive thought was.

_____

_____

_____

# Working Together

Working together is an important part of being a good friend. Read the following situations. Write down how the people can work together to solve the problems.

**Situation 1: The playground is covered in trash.**

How can the students work together to solve this problem?

_____

_____

**Situation 2: Pasta spilled all over the kitchen floor.**

How can the family work together to solve this problem?

_____

_____

**Situation 3: One friend is feeling left out of the handball game.**

How can the friends work together to solve this problem?

_____

_____

Your friend says they don't want a hug. What is another way you can show them you care without touching them?

_____

_____

_____

Imagine your friend told you they were feeling lonely. Your friend wants your advice about how they can feel better. What would you say to them?

_____

_____

_____

Why is it important to listen when other people are talking?

_____

_____

_____

# Helping Our Ocean Friends

Draw a picture of the ocean. Draw a picture of all the animals living in the ocean that we help by cleaning up our trash.

Have you ever felt left out by your friends? What is something you can say to tell your friends how you feel when you are left out?

_____

_____

_____

Imagine you are part of a pack of wolves. One of the other wolves has a hurt foot. What can you do to help the hurt wolf?

_____

_____

_____

Why is it important to share your toys?

_____

_____

_____

## Acts of Kindness

We can show our friends and family we care in lots of ways. We can listen to them, offer them a hug, or spend time with them. Write down ways you can show kindness this week.

**How I will be kind to a parent or trusted adult:**

_____
_____

**How I will be kind to a friend:**

_____
_____

**How I will be kind to my pet or an animal:**

_____
_____

**How I will be kind to the environment:**

_____
_____

Have you ever worked with a friend on a project? What made it hard? What made it easy?

_____

_____

_____

What should your face be doing when you are listening to your teacher?

_____

_____

_____

What are two ways you can show someone you are listening when they are talking?

_____

_____

_____

# SUPERPOWER PRACTICE: LISTENING IS MY SUPERPOWER!

Listening is an important part of showing our friends and family we care. This week, try using the listening skills listed here and check them off as you do them.

- ☐ Look at a person when they are talking.
- ☐ Nod your head.
- ☐ Smile or make a kind face.
- ☐ Don't walk around or move a lot.
- ☐ Do not talk when other people are talking.

**Bonus!** How do you know when someone is listening carefully to you? How does it make you feel?

_____

_____

_____

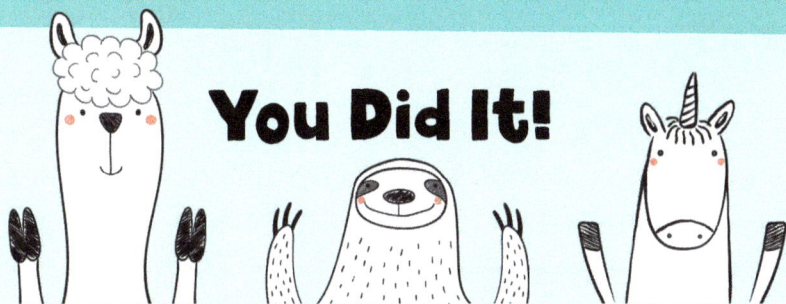

# You Did It!

Congratulations! You did it! Thank you for working hard and being thoughtful as you filled in your empathy journal. You have completed your journal and built empathy skills. You learned that empathy means feeling or understanding what other people are feeling. You learned listening skills, caring skills, and how to be kind to everyone around you. You practiced calming your body and showing respect to others.

The skills you learned in this journal will help you become the best friend you can be. Even though your empathy journal is done, your empathy and kindness journey continues!

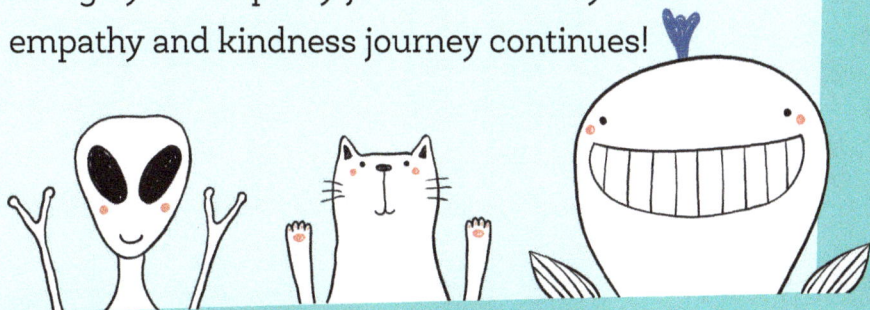

# Resources for Kids

*Empathy Is Your Superpower: A Book About Understanding the Feelings of Others*
by Cori Bussolari
This book is a fun story with activities to continue practicing your empathy skills.

*It's Brave to Be Kind: A Kindness Book for Children That Teaches Empathy and Compassion*
by Natasha Daniels
Check out this book for even more help practicing kindness.

*Me and My Feelings: A Kids' Guide to Understanding and Expressing Themselves*
by Vanessa Green Allen
We all have big feelings! This book will help you explore all your feelings and share them with others.

# Resources for Grown-Ups

*Mindfulness Journal for Parents: Prompts and Practices to Stay Calm, Present, and Connected*
by Josephine Atluri
This is a handy journal with prompts and exercises to help you stay calm and work through moments of stress with your child.

*Rethinking Discipline: Conscious Parenting Strategies for Growth and Connection*
by Yehudis Smith
This book offers a practical guide to conscious parenting with simple, effective strategies.

## About the Author

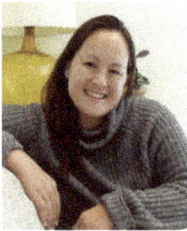

**Kelley Stevens** is a licensed marriage and family therapist in Santa Barbara, California. Kelley specializes in working with kids, teens, and families. When she isn't working with clients, she enjoys hanging out with her toddler and puppy!

www.ingramcontent.com/pod-product-compliance
Lightning Source LLC
Chambersburg PA
CBHW042047050426
42452CB00019BA/2963